The Journey Continues...

By Cheri Ann Revill

ISBN:1505922038
ISBN-13:9781505922035

DEDICATION

To all my teachers thank you for your lessons for without
them I would not be who I am today!

CONTENTS

LIFE

You are sitting on your couch
thinking about life
What are you going to do?
Where is it taking you?
Nothing is going to change
You are as miserable as can be
What if you could change it?
It is that simple you will see
Have a look around you
and maybe you will find
That maybe it's not so bad
I am breathing, well aren't I?
So what can I do
to make a difference somehow
to make life a little easier
a little happier, have more joy for me and mine?
So get off that couch
Go and walk outside
Have a look at mother earth
and see what you can find
Someone walks past
and smiles and says Hello

Maybe just maybe there is another way to go!

By Cheri Ann Revill

Prelude

In the days that follow, there are fleeting moments of loneliness, but they are gone like the wind, for we are truly not alone in the sense of our true presence. We are surrounded by others who are always there guiding, protecting, healing and loving. So stop and be, listen and feel, feel with your heart, with your being and you will sense that someone maybe there watching over you. Yes, the physical being craves touch, the human body loves to be touched and nurtured through physical love. There is a whole new sense of being when we feel on another level. Feel the wind caress your skin, feel the heat from the sun on your body, on a beautiful summers day. The sand underneath your feet, between your toes, the ocean, and the seawater engulf you as you dive under the waves. The trees whisper to you through their leaves and branches as you walk by, the flowers follow you, as you smell their scent. We are touched everywhere we go by nature, mother earth and how she cares for us. Like most of our mothers did when we were infants and do we not long for our mother's touch, her hug, her kiss as we did when we were young and from that we knew everything would be all right. As I sit here writing this, I hear the sounds, of the birds, the insects, the wind and other elements of the earth surround me. I feel their presence within me and know I am never truly alone. What will you do? Where will you go? What are your dreams and aspirations? What would you like to do with your life whilst you are here for this lifetime? It could be something as simple as being Happy! It could be, being a good parent, to touch someone's life? Change the world? Are you living your dream? What are you doing to make it happen? What have you asked for?

What have you put into place? I was always doing, from sunup to sundown. Children, husband, cleaning, shopping, cooking, working, pets, studying. There was always something to do. It has taken me awhile to be able to just sit and do nothing because if I did that, I felt lazy! Even now I don't sit for too long, but I do sit. Sometimes it could be even going for a walk, a stroll, somewhere that gives you peace! Where ever it takes you, to help you still your mind, stop thinking for a few minutes, listen, feel and look around you. Take in every precious second of what is going on in that moment, stop, don't think, stop, sense, feel! What happens? Anything? Nothing? No wrong or right here. What to do now? Where to go? What do I want my life to look like? Where do I want to go? What do I want to do? Yes, you may have commitments, jobs, families and so on. Could it be easier, happier? What would that look like for you? Ask the question and see what happens! Make a choice, don't like it, make another choice, no right or wrong all you have to do is choose. Some things are out of your control. No point worrying about it, so give it up, let it go, it will always work out in the end, maybe even better than you think it would, all you have to do is believe. What do you know? Do you know that everything will always work out? Do you believe that everything will be Ok? It's a good belief and knowing that will happen is even better, trusting that it will, is the icing on top! Always know the best possible outcome will happen, go one better and know, believe and trust that everything will work out way better than you could ever imagine! Wouldn't that be awesome? Ask for the impossible, anything is possible. There is more than enough for everyone in this world, so why not put it out there to the universe what you would like, your desires, your dreams.

Then when ideas come into your head of possibilities or someone comes along and gives you an idea, run with it, you never know where it will take you. Believe in you, know that anything is possible and you will be surprised of what comes about. Be patient though, this is one I am learning every day, it will happen, it may not happen how you think it is going to happen, but it will. When, where and how it happens is not for us to figure out just know it will and it will! I believe in the Law of Attraction, your thoughts become feelings and those feelings become reality.

So be careful what you put out there because you will always attract it.

THE WALK

You set out for your walk, one step at a time.
You start to ascend finding beauty on either side of
you,
One step at a time.
As you get higher the ground becomes rockier,
maneuvering each step with care and grace over
each rock,
One step at a time.
Here it flattens out, the grass is green and lush,
you look up to find beautiful trees all around,
birds flitting about,
you take a deep breath and continue up,
One step at a time.
The climb becomes steeper, your breathing becomes
shallow,
you can do it,
One step at a time.
Then it comes to that point you feel you can not go
on,
there is pain from within, but you are so close only a
few more,
so you push on,

One step at a time.

You go over the last ridge, you are there, you look up

and the view is magnificent.

Your breathing starts to slow as you take in the

beauty all around you,

The pain is forgotten, there are no words to express

what you see.

I am so grateful I made it,

I am grateful for the view,

I am grateful I could do it,

One step at a time.

Life is like the walk,

it all depends on you,

you can do anything,

all you have to do is know that

you can do.

So go on, make that choice, make it now, all you have

to do is take that first step and take,

ONE STEP AT A TIME.

By Cheri Ann Revill

More of My Story

The perception of life, love, happiness, anything really comes from so many different angles. Culture, religion, spirituality, socio-economic regions/levels, countries, beliefs, faiths, governments and family structures. These perceptions shape each individuals life and some are so ingrained it becomes second nature. There would be no need to change any part of their life because they see nothing wrong with it! Then comes the judgmental side where others voice their opinions because they do not understand another individual's way of life, their choices, and their beliefs. In my experience, change only comes from either a place of darkness, pain, suffering and the decision never ever to go through that again stems the fight for change. Not accepting the norm, there is more to life than what everyone has excepted and the individual has decided to make every opportunity there is to change the outcome of their life. Then there is the deep seeded notion that you just know there is more to life, something better out there. Life is not meant to be this difficult, relationships are not meant to be this hard, surely I deserve to be Happy?

This was the place I came from to make the changes I wanted to become happier! I knew from early in my life there was an easier way of doing things... there had to be more to my life, more to me and why did Love elude me to how I felt I should be loved! I thought I was unlovable, as I was told often enough, that I started to believe it! Yet I tried many different self help tools, counseling to get me through my every day life, I even would run away at times, to come back and cope for a little bit longer. The vow was what kept me in place, the expectations of me, myself. 'I had made my bed now I have to lie in it'. So until that decision was made for me, I will be eternally grateful for that decision. After grieving for a period of time I realised it was an actual blessing, I was FREE! I was actually free to live my life my way, something I had not experienced before and so the journey begins, which became very exciting.

Slowing down, removing the stress from my body, my health was my first priority and the start of healing my body had begun. It took me about two years too learn to slow down, that meant stop studying, no working, being a mum and finding me!

Now for me this was quite a challenge as I had literally worked since I can remember. Even as a child, homework had to be perfect and there was always extra study, physical activity was a daily structure. From the age of seven we had to run around the block or as soon as we had learnt to swim, we had to do laps so we were always doing something. By the time I turned 16, I was given the choice to stop swimming training, I did! Grades and sport was a good way to receive my father's approval and love. When I thought that wasn't working I started to do the normal teenage things.

When my father became ill with Cancer when I was 23, only then was I able to let him know how I felt. Mum actually came up to me and asked me to apologise to him about everything I had done, I was outraged, then and there I vowed to tell them how I really felt. I wrote it down and read it to them, they had no idea and after a week or so they read to me how sorry they were and how much they loved me and was extremely proud of me. I am so grateful that happened, though it still took years of counseling to help me shift the grief and anger that I felt and acknowledge that how I was treated was not the norm. I knew I wanted to parent my children differently, but if you don't deal with your own feelings they seem to come out somewhere else! I find that now more than ever, by learning to love me, put me first I am a better mother, kinder, have more patience and be more loving.

Control, we all have parts of our life we want to control, be it our bodies, our relationships, work place, children and family. We like to feel we have control, to give us that sense of achievement. Do we really? Do we really have any control over anything? We like to think we do, but how often does it work out perfectly? We plan how things are supposed to be, how others are meant to act and it never actually happens. We are so disappointed, we become angry or frustrated and we either blame everyone else or everything else for it going so horribly wrong! Some even go into the wrongness of them that they are not good enough, can never get anything right, they are useless. What if we gave up that control, maybe control is an illusion? We may know the outcome of a few things and maybe the rest is up to fate! If we gave up that control, would life not be easier?

Less worrying and stress, all that time wasted on something we had no control over. We could be enjoying our daily lives with the things that make us happy! There was a time, I was guilty of doing something similar, trying to control members of my family because that is what I thought would make my life easier. In my experience, I found this is not the case! From a time that I can remember as a child my father would control me through fear, fear of him getting mad and then I would be in trouble. As the years progressed I started to stand up to him and he would start to hit me, so then I would be submissive to his way of doing things. Now I thought this was normal, as I had heard from other kids that they all got smacked in one form of another. It wasn't until I was going to counseling with my eldest son for his anger, that I was informed that I was actually being beaten. It just wasn't a smack on the backside, I was belted around the head or with a belt around the bottom half of me. This took a while to sink in as I knew it was not how I wanted to bring up my own children and I had to relearn a different style of parenting which took a number of years.

As I grew and left home, the Army was not much
different than home funny enough, but new ways of
control were substituted. A few months into basic
training I was in trouble for things teenagers get up to
(underage drinking etc.) and two of us were being
made examples of. Our punishments were a little
harsher than usual and we were also threatened with
prison! For any 17 year old this would be a frightening
experience and I thought there was no way out. I had
no idea what to do, where to go or who to turn too! A
higher-ranking soldier propositioned me and in return
I was promised, I would not go to prison. What do I
do? I knew it wasn't right but felt I had no choice.
Years later I realised it was a form of rape, control
over another where there is no way out for the other
party. I always thought rape would be the worse thing
for a woman to go through but I regarded that as a
violent act. This I found out was not the case as it
happened again years later, when a man I thought
was a friend came into the house, forced himself onto
me and said that he could have his way whenever he
wished. For over twenty years I thought it was my
own fault that I somehow provoked him and it was all

my own doing. Two years ago, I accepted that it wasn't and it was rape. Through out my life I have been physically and emotionally abused in one form or another, not realizing it until it was too late. These were some of the ways that control was used against me. Maybe they felt threatened, felt inadequate or that was the only way they knew how! I accept responsibility for all of it, I gave over my power, to them, to keep the peace, to take the path of least resistance. When I did this, I took back my power and said no more!

This does not work for me, I deserve better, if you don't like me, if you don't love me than that is your issue not mine. It is not me, there is nothing wrong with me, I am beautiful, I am smart, I can do or be anything. That is when things really started to change!

LOVE

Love is different for many

Love has many words and actions

Love can be shown from within

Love can be in the darkest of places

Love is unique for most

Love is seen everywhere

Love has a variety of scenes

Love has been shown somewhere

Love is for the mighty

Love is for the meek

Love is the greatest emotion

Love is what we seek

Love is wished for by everyone

Love can be felt by all

In truth Love is within you and makes you stand

straight and tall.

By Cheri Ann Revill

My New Body

As I found my body starting to shift and change, lose weight, everything changed! I gave up control over my body and what I would like it to look like, from size, shape, age, colour everything! Body you look how you would like to look, how you are supposed to look. I let go of all points of views and judgment that I picked up about my body, consciously and subconsciously. I started to listen and take the time to learn to love me again. Over a two year period I lost weight, a lot of weight, my hair colour changed, with a slight curl (where I had always had straight hair), my skin complexion changed, my eyes became clearer and brighter. I was healthier and the changes continued, all from learning to listen to my body and giving up that control. How my body would like to move changes often, but I still love walking along the beach. There are dietary changes every week for what ever my body requires to help itself to heal and how it would love to look! Going with these changes may seem too difficult for some as they don't like change but for me I would rather feel and look amazing and love my body, then go back to how I felt before.

Listening to your body is a daily regime, it is now a part of my life and with each new day it becomes easier and easier.

How you are feeling in my experience, is a very important factor of creating a life of happiness. Not only does it change your body from the inside out but your life in general. The relief of stress from your body, is a key component of healing your body completely and that is done by being aware of how you are feeling throughout your day. How you feel, will help with changing your thought process. What you are thinking creates how you feel, if you are feeling good your thoughts are good ones and if you are feeing not so good, your thoughts correlate with that feeling.

This is a great way to monitor your thoughts through your feelings and it will help change your thoughts from negative ones to more positive ones. Thinking of something that brings a smile to your face, a piece of music, a good memory, funny movie or doing something that you love to do, will give you those good feelings. I have found, for me, saying Thank you over and over again, helps shift the thoughts as it distracts me from what I was thinking. I then find things that I am grateful for, I look at what I do have and I feel truly blessed.

You have to work at changing your thought processes every day. When you wake up think wonderful thoughts, be grateful for another day, for a great sleep in a bed, that you are breathing easily and think about what wonderful adventures you will have that day. No matter if you are going to work, or you have to get the kids ready, caring for a loved one, start each day with positive thoughts and have a wonderful feeling within and watch the day unfurl into an amazing day.

Being grateful is not just words, saying Thank you because you think you have to be polite.

Being grateful comes from a much deeper place of feeling, it's heartfelt.

Having gratitude is life changing, you know how truly blessed you are, to have beauty surround you every day. To have the privileges that keep you in a state of comfort, the life that comes in the form of your body, the people who surround you, the love you feel for yourself and others, there is so much that one takes for granted.

Without these things a difference surely would be

noticed!

You feel grateful with every cell of your being, which leaves no room for complaints, worry or stress.

Your belief, your faith and your gratitude, as you know the Universe has got everything covered. I am not saying there won't be bumps through-out the day, but it is up to you, how you react to those hiccups. Change your views, your perceptions, on how you see those 'problems' and different solutions will come to mind or they may solve themselves, you never know what may happen. Look at the words you use every day, this is hard, miserable, can't do it, sick, it's impossible. Try to change them to the opposite word, this is easy, I can, anything is possible, wonderful, healthy and so on, watch how it makes a difference in your life.

My whole day has then been changed because I changed my thoughts, which then changed my feelings, or you could say it changed my mood! Learning to notice how you feel will get easier the more you do it and then you will find you have more good days than bad.

Do what makes you happy. Find something that you can do every day that makes you happy and this will also help change your perception of your life. By doing these things your body will feel so much better, you will be more aware of your body's needs and be able to help your body to heal itself as it is meant to. You will have more energy, as stress uses a lot of the body's energy, that is why you find you are tired all the time. Other benefits will be your health improves, you may notice how your look changes and you look forward to each day with renewed hope! Having a healthy love for yourself can change so many aspects of your body not only on the inside but on the outside as well. Listen to what your body may require to help with this process, be intuned with your bodies needs, movement, rest, food, vitamins, minerals and any other therapies it may need.

Since I have started this journey, I have been to a chiropractor which helped aligned my posture, which in turn helped my nervous system improve, helping my whole body. I have had acupuncture to help reduce the excess skin and for it to fit over my body again as it should, without surgery. Different kinds of massages, different kinds of movement, walking, yoga and swimming. Now my body has completely changed through listening, being intuned with it, helping its healing process, not only have I lost an incredible amount of weight. I look younger, my skin looks amazing, my eyes are clear and bright, my hair colour has changed (I have not coloured my hair for nearly two years), and all the sickness I used to endure every year I no longer have. The benefits I have encountered since I started, have definitely outweighed, every other reason not to do it, there is no looking back. Now I am developing these tools to use in other areas of my life, to create a better life for my children and myself.

Patience for me has been one of the most challenging aspects out of this whole process. Even though I have improved immensely since I began my journey, it still gets the better of me as I wish to have it all yesterday. You do have to be patient, not only with your self but also the results, as you want it to be done with ease. If your body is not physically ready for the change that is going on within you, it can become very uncomfortable. I know this from experience because when I started I said what ever it takes I am changing! Never again will I say this, I always say with ease now! The easier it is, the quicker it will happen, now that may seem to be quite odd but if you push before your body is ready or even if you are not ready mentally, it becomes challenging and the process takes longer.

If you are not at the stage of thinking and believing in yourself, any changes that are made may not stay that way. For many individuals who have gone to lose any amount of weight or try to change how they look, most of the time they either put the weight back on or keep going back for more and more changes. For if you haven't learnt to love who you are and believe in yourself, you will fall back into your old way of thinking, therefore always seeing yourself how you used to look.

This would have to be the most important factor in this whole process, learn to like, then love you, believe in you and when the changes happen they are more likely to stay that way or even be more than you ever thought possible.

I know I was blown away and many people don't even

recognise me now. Be patient, it will happen when it happens, there is a saying, that you get it when you get it! There is no right or wrong, there is no time limit if you don't get it by this time there is something wrong with you!

NO! That is not the case, we are all different, we all understand things differently, we see everything differently, be patient with yourself, be gentle with yourself, believe you can do it and anything is possible and watch what happens!

FRIENDSHIPS

Friendships are bound together

In many shapes and forms

from fleeting moments

to years of togetherness

Friendships are formed with the strongest of bonds

and some friendships are broken as easily as a

spider's web.

No matter how many or how few

Over the period of a lifetime

We will have many different kinds of friendships

Some we Love like family, others are acquaintances

How many we have or how they are formed, is

irrelevant

As they all teach us valuable lessons through out our

life

Whether we see them in that moment or years from

now

We will always remember the friendships

We have had for many years to come.

By Cheri Ann Revill

Living

When I thought the life I knew was coming to an end.
It was actually the beginning of something wonderful!
There the journey begins, which became very
exciting.

Happiness is a choice. Once you have made a
decision about anything in your life, then it is easy to
follow through. You just have to take that first step
and that is to make a choice! What do you want to
be? How do you want to live this life? How do you
want to feel on a daily basis?

To choose, to decide what it is you really want, it may
be difficult but it will be the greatest gift you ever give
yourself. You will be then putting your needs before
others, your dreams, are important too, your life is
your own no one else can do it for you. Own it take
responsibility for yourself and make a choice. Taking
responsibility for your life, for everything that happens
in your life, is a monumental step! Yes everything that
has happened to you up to this point be responsible
for it and everything that happens to you today and
every day after, you have consciously or

subconsciously asked for.

If you don't like it change it and yes it is that simple. All you have to do is make that decision, make a different choice and believe you deserve to have the life you have always dreamed of.

Life is what you make it! Isn't that what they say? I would say that is true. In my experience the life you lead, you have chosen, wanted or asked for in some way or another and if it is not then why have you not changed it? Why have you not chosen something different something you would like, to do, to be, to have! At some point you have to take responsibility for yourself, for your life.

Forget about what has been, you can not do anything about that now, you have today and the rest of your life.

Why not do it? You don't like change, it worries you, it even scares you! Fear is what stops most people from choosing something different, fear of the unknown, they need to know how it is going to all work out.

There are responsibilities, family, bills, where to live, how to survive? Yes there is all of that but if you put it into place that you have made the decision to have that sea change, choose where you want to live, look at work or maybe you would like to do something completely different!

Go back and study, work for yourself.

Buy a new home or rent, find a new job, new schools you never know it may be the best decision, choice, you ever make. If you never try you will never know. General Happiness, one sense of self, living life to its fullest, being love, feeling love, gratitude, its the expectations I have found to be our downfall. The expectations we have on ourselves and others that are really quite high.

Why do we have any expectations at all? For me I grew up on your word is your bond.

If you say you are going to do something you do it! If you are unable to do it due to unforeseen circumstances then be honest about it and tell them. If you plan on not doing anything then don't say anything. Disappointment and mistrust in people is high on the list of why very little is done for others. There is an expectation that if you do something for another you expect something in return! How does that make you feel? If there is no expectations, if you give for the joy of giving, the sense of fulfillment within yourself, a sense of purpose, filled with love is that not a gift in itself?

I have found in my experience, that even when it comes to the little things within a family unit, doing for your partner, your children, siblings, parents, there is an expectation of, 'if I do this for you then I expect you to do the same for me'! I have learnt this lesson many times over, and have been disappointed on many occasions! I have realised that they are not me. They don't think like me, feel like me and view life the way I do. So how in the world are they going to do the same as me when it comes to giving to me? Give up all expectations, give up their perception of you, your perception of them!

If you want to do something for another then do it with no expectations of getting something in return. You do it because that is what you do, you enjoy it, it gives you a satisfaction, joy, brings you happiness. Don't do it because you feel you have to, do it because you want to.

What are you doing that no longer work's for you? What are you doing that you have been doing for so long that you do it out of habit? It could be something that you no longer like doing? Anything that doesn't feel good anymore?

There are many different perceptions on what letting go means to an individual.

Firstly for me it was to stop living in the past and to let go everything that had happened that still affected me. Forgiving those who I felt had caused me hurt and pain, though they may never even known that they had, was a process I had to go through. Then forgiving myself, this is a whole different realm of processing. It means accepting responsibility for everything that has happened, the choices I made and to stop blaming myself for them. For some it may be hard to get your head around this idea, though in my experience this helped me to let go of all that happened in the past, the physical, and emotional abuse I had suffered, to change myself knowing that it will never happen again! How do you change your self so that it doesn't happen again? You may have seen people go into the same types of relationships time and again that don't work out and then they think there is something wrong with them. The choices they make are because of the way they feel about them selves. So to change how you feel about yourself you need to look at yourself in a different light and by doing that you need to wipe all that has happened in the past and start again.

Look at yourself from within, what do you like about yourself, what don't you like and why? The judgments you have about yourself, you have seen, been told or heard them somewhere along the line and taken them on board as truth. Learn to like yourself, like your company, if you don't like your own company how can someone else enjoy your company? Love yourself, like you would like others to love you? It is something you have to work at every day and in my experience it has worked for me, it took some time but I got there eventually!

I didn't like my own company I didn't love me for who I was and once I started to do that everything else changed, how I looked, how I was treated by others and life in general! Looking at how I thought, the words I used, giving up control of things that I never had control over to begin with! What will be will be, and always have your best foot forward, look on the brighter side of life. Yes it does make a difference on your outlook of the world, life, yourself, and others! You put just as much energy into positive and as you do the negative thoughts.

Which outcomes would you prefer? I would rather have a happy, easy approach to life than the other way around.

Yes it is possible. Anything is possible if you believe it enough!

Control, we all have parts of our life we want to control, be it, our bodies, our relationships, work place, children, family. We like to feel we have control, to give us that sense achievement. But do we really? Do we really have any control over anything? We like to think we do, but how often does it work out perfectly?

We plan how things are supposed to be, how others are meant to act and does it actually happen. We are so disappointed, or we get angry, frustrated and we either blame everyone else or everything else. Some even go into the wrongness of them, that they are not good enough, can never get anything right, they are useless. What if we gave up that control, maybe control is an illusion. There are only very few things we know the out-come of and the rest is up to fate? If we gave up that control, would life not be easier, not so much worrying, stress, all that time wasted on something we had no control over, where we could have been enjoying our daily lives with the things that made us happy!

BELIEVE

What do you believe in?

Do you believe the grass is green, the sky is blue?

The air all around us is what keeps us true!

Do you believe that true love will conquer all?

or Love is how we crack apart and fall.

Do you believe the earth is round?

or the earth is a mess and will come crashing down.

Do you believe there is something for all of us in this
life?

or that we all are set in our ways and nothing will
prepare us for the fight.

Do you believe that there are many possibilities?

or there is no way out and people have no creativity.

Do you believe that when all else fails, everything will
be OK?

Maybe it will, or maybe it will just stay that way.

Do you believe in you?

Why would I do that, I am never going to go out and
play

What do you Believe in?

Me I believe in me,

I believe that the possibilities are endless

I believe the earth and her inhabitants will be saved

I believe in Happiness and Love

I believe that people can change

Not only do I believe in Me but I believe in YOU too!

By Cheri Ann Revill

Believable

Believable or unbelievable? This is up to the individual of what they want to believe. What has changed their perception on an event to change their belief system! I have always known that the body was capable of so much more, hence my interest in biology of the human body. Yet I believed all that I had been told since I was young and it wasn't until I was at university and learning about the diseases, symptoms and what medications to use to help with the symptoms of the disease.

I thought there had to be a better way, than putting a band aid (covering up) the underlying issues that create the disease in the first place! With my own history of dealing with stress, depression, skin issues and other ailments that affected my family, and myself I realised that the thought processes, in one form or another, were the reason why we got sick. Now that may sound pretty incredible, why would we want to be sick, some more serious than others, the pain, the discomfort and everything else that comes with it. Look at the humble cold, every year everyone seems to get a cold and react to it.

In the sense when someone gets a cold they react in saying, 'everyone in the family is now going to get a cold' or in the classroom, day care, work and everyone expresses how they spread germs to everyone's else. Germs are very real yes, but we can choose to spread them or not. Consciously and subconsciously we have accepted that we are going to get a cold every year, the flu, its flu season, so we are going to get the flu! What if we changed how we thought? What if this year you make the decision, I am healthy, completely healthy, no colds, no flu, no sickness at all? This may be quite strange because it has been inbuilt in us since we were born! Have you heard, if you are cold you will catch a cold, if the baby is sick, mum will get sick or if a sibling is sick now the baby will get sick! It seems to become a vicious circle because we have projected this within ourselves, which has become solidified, into our bodies. We are so focused on becoming sick with something that we are always justified when it does, 'I knew it', or 'see I told you'. Our body is capable of so much more than we are led to believe that if we believed it, it would change the way we live completely.

Your body was made from a single cell and from that cell it has the ability to create a whole new body within a matter of a few years and has the ability to heal itself too! Believe, Listen, Love and be grateful for our bodies, we can completely transform them into an amazing physical form, even how we look! Yes, age has a lot to do with it, as we have accepted that we will age a certain way and we will have certain ailments due to what age we are. What if that was not the case at all? What if we didn't look how may years we are, as it is only a number?

What if we could live to double the age that has been expected or more, still being able to do everything we are meant to do? I believe in all of this and more! I have done this, I am completely healthy, and I have transformed my body without surgery and I look younger! Yes it is possible, anything is possible if you believe it. To remove all points of view and judgment from your body, may take some time. You have a lifetime of beliefs solidified within your body. Remove all stress from your life, be happy, love yourself, be grateful for your amazing body, listen to what your body would like to eat and drink, which is an ongoing process that I do every day! Be patient with yourself and over time you will notice the transformation occur. Believe in yourself is a fundamental basis of Law of Attraction. You need to trust yourself, believe in yourself, know anything is possible and believe it with your entire being. It doesn't matter how, when, or why just know that it will! The universe and your body will sort out the rest. Think about your Dream, feel that you already have it and how wonderful it makes you feel. Picture it like a dream, picture yourself doing, being that dream!

Now do the same with your body, picture yourself how you would like to look and believe that it is possible. Never lose faith, hope, don't waver in your thoughts, that it will never happen, hold onto it tight and watch the miracle unfurl.
You may have things happen, helping you go in the right direction, that is where your intuition plays a big part.
If it feels good/right do it, if it doesn't don't!
Yes it is as simple as that, not enough of us listen and

use our intuition, especially on a daily basis. It is there showing us the way to our happiness.

Yes believing in yourself is the start of a great adventure, which will bring the extraordinary into your life, more than you could ever imagine. Believing that I could write, let alone a book was mind boggling to me but that was the direction I was given. I had no idea of what I wanted to do, all I knew was, I love teaching, public speaking and helping others.

I started writing a journal of how I felt, my experiences daily and a gratitude journal. Then I went to writing quotes for my Facebook page, that inspired me and hopefully others, and then it was poetry.

After a while I found that if I didn't over think it, the words would flow as I wrote and the next thing you know I had enough to put a book together! With the encouragement from others, who read my writings, it helped me to continue and gave me the confidence to publish my books and the rest is history.

As I look back it was what I asked for because it suited me as I was going through life changes.

Looking after my children and learning to love me, find my happiness and where I want to be, what I wanted my life to look like.

It may not look like how I thought it would or show up how I thought it was going to, I just knew it would and it did! Trust, believe and receive all, know it to be true, know all your needs will be met, you will always have more than enough, be positive, think less and enjoy life, be grateful, have fun and Love.

The subconscious mind is your thoughts that have solidified into your entire being in other words you have believed them to be your truth, had them often and now they are part of you! You can change this, it may take time and you also may have forgotten all about these because it has been years since you have believed that thought process to be your truth. Your body will react to the thoughts that you have over this lifetime from a child to this present moment. From how you will age, to how you will die, to relationships, money anything really, you had already decided and it is all locked up into your body.

How do you change this? How do you remove them from your body? Letting go of all points of views and judgments that you had on any particular subject and rewriting how you would like it to be. A good place to start is before you fall asleep think of a different way of being, what you would like your life to look like, how you would love to feel and how healthy would you like your body to be. This is where your conscious mind is overridden and your thoughts will go straight to your subconscious. Remember be careful with what you wish for, negative or positive, if you put enough thought, energy and time into it, you will receive it. Make sure you know what it is you want and think of how you are going to word it! It does take time but if you want it badly enough keep going and be grateful for what you have so more or better will show up.

Everything is what we see, we are all a part of it, we are all connected, we are all one, the billions of atoms, the vibrations of energy that make up everything in this universe. We can create, manifest anything we desire if we are of the same vibration, of what we would like to create!
Everything else doesn't matter, it is insignificant, all the little things we worry about, which has nothing to do with us. Our intent, our focus is to feel good, be Happy, feel joy, be grateful, feel bliss and focus on

our intent of what we would like our life to be!

This is how we create the lives we live so if we want to change it believe we can and it shall be so.

FLY

Watching the birds from inside, you see them dancing
You watch them chirp and sing to one another
Then they take flight, going this way and that way
Going from one tree to the next, back down to the
ground
One takes off soaring into the blue sky and you watch
until it is but a speck in the distance
That is when you stand and walk outside, the birds all
scatter to the wind
No matter, you have taken in their message to you
You can also sing your song, take flight and explore
One day when you are able, knowing you will be
strong enough
You will also spread your wings and soar into the
great unknown
Knowing that now your adventure called Life has
begun.

By Cheri Ann Revill

Patience and Trust

How do you find yourself after being married, becoming a mother at the age of 18, a grandmother and a mother again for the last time at the age of 40? A very good question, which I asked myself! Who am I and what is it exactly do I want out of life? What did I want my life to look like? What is happiness and love to me? Where do you start? For me the best place to start was to start with me! I had a really good look at myself and realised I didn't like myself, didn't even like being a woman!

I found that being a woman seemed to make it even more difficult to get anywhere in this life than it already was! How do you turn that around? I had to change my thought processes, by looking at myself as an amazon princess. It was Ok to be feminine, be strong, independent and beautiful. With everything I had achieved in my life so far, it was credible I just had to believe it and over time I did. I looked at everything I was doing at the time, which parts did I do because I enjoyed it or because of the responsibly of being a mother and a wife?

As I was no longer a wife, all of the points of views and judgments I had about that, I could now let go. Being a mother on the other hand I had basically started again, I had two adult children and two children under the age of six. Looking at my older boys logically, I was no longer responsible for them, they could make their own choices, live their own lives. All I had to do was to love them and support them in all their endeavours. During this process the one thing I did learn is that my happiness impacted on my children, if I was happy with who I am, with my life, they would be happy too!

It also made me a better mother, no longer stressed, so particular with everything, worrying about what other people thought. That was a major hurdle for me, as a young mother I was told I would not be a good mum and I was striving to be just that, to no avail in my eyes, that is! Learning to like yourself you realise that most of your judgements about yourself, are unfounded and once you are able to let go of them it feels like that the weight of the world has been lifted from your shoulders.

I started to look for what I wanted my life to look like,

what did I want to do, where did I want to live?

I really didn't want to be at university, as what I knew was not being reflected in my marks. You have to write like they want you to write, learn certain parts of the subject matter by knowing either procedures or wording of particular processes! Whether you knew how to do it, understood the subject, did not matter! In my experience this was not preparing you for the real world as they said they were. I didn't like living in the city, noise, sirens, smell, sadness it was quite depressing!

There and then I decided that I would defer my university degree and move to the beach.

Once that decision was made it took six months for it all to fall into place. I love it! The other thing that was quite a challenge for me was spending time with myself, as I did not like myself, why would I want to spend time with me! That was an adventure let me tell you, now that took some time, years even! Where as now I enjoy my alone time, I take the time to do the things I love to do. I go for the long walks along the beach, go out for coffee, I take myself out on a date, dinner and a movie.

Potter around the house or in the garden, go

shopping, write, which I never thought I would enjoy so much!

I am still learning about the things I love to do and I have the rest of my life to find out. Learning to love yourself is quite a journey and once you start, you become curious as to what else there is about you, you never knew. That feeling that you enjoy your company, you look good even better than good and all of those years where you were told that you never measured up, what were they on about! You find it doesn't matter what other people think, you don't even care anymore because you know that within you, you are happy with who you are, you love who you are and that is all that matters!

Patience and trust, trust that it will happen and be patient it will happen when it is ready not when you are. It will not happen overnight, it does take time and you have to work at it everyday. Like any habit, to break it, it takes a conscious effort on a daily basis. There are years of thought processes, beliefs, judgments, points of views to shift, so that you can change them to what you would like to believe, not what the general population of the world believes in!

You need to be patient with yourself there is no right

or wrong, you do the very best that you can do on any particular day.

Then start again, the next day and then the next until it requires no effort at all, it is inbuilt and it comes with ease. In my experience, I am now aware of how I am feeling through my thoughts and I have a chance to change that feeling by changing my thoughts! I choose to feel good through being happy, having unconditional love for myself, others and the world around me, also by being grateful for all that I have, be and see every day.

This helped take the focus off what I thought was not going right. The negative that is in the world and the doubt that may creep in from time to time.

Having unwavering faith that everything is going to turn out way better than I could ever expect, follow my dreams, no matter how they will come true, just know that they will! Dreams yes dreams, do you have any dreams, what are your desires? Change your focus on what is going wrong, what you don't have and find the dream you would love to have, to live, look at what you do have and be grateful for those things.

Listen to the words that are being spoken by you and others, life is hard, I can't do this, I hate, debt, sickness all of these seem to be in general conversation these days!

What happened to all the wonderful things, happy things, positive things that happen every day in the world around us? If you focus on more of those things, talk about all the wonderful positive things that are going on in your life, you will notice a difference in how you live your life, how you view life and so on.

Now this may be a challenge to start with, it will take some practice because it seems to be ingrained in how we talk to each other these days. Another thing if others choose to have conversations about their health issues, money trouble, relationship hassles etc. try not to take them on board. Change the subject into something a little bit lighter, positive, it may help change their point of view, even their mood! It may not either way you may not feel so drained when you walk away from the conversation.

I have stopped reading the papers, magazines, listening to the news, current affair programs, as you seem to be reeled into all the negative stuff that is happening in the world.

I found it a challenge to shift how I was feeling after watching or reading current events, as it all seemed to be overwhelming with negative news.

Shifting back into feeling good was quite a struggle, therefore I stopped listening to it all together. If I needed to know anything I would find out from other people!

For me, feeling good is a priority as it helps me to manifest the wonderful life I live, the amazing body I have and for me this is more important than all the negative that seems to be talked about every minute of every day!

I choose happiness and ease in my life, in my children's life, as I only have now to enjoy this amazing gift that I have been given! As the journey continues so do the new and wonderful experiences we have the opportunity of having. The people we meet that touch our lives in so many ways. The lessons that we learn and the gratitude we feel for having known them, no matter for how long. Throughout our lives we have met hundreds of people, even thousands and each one of them has touched us in some way.

They have played a part in shaping and moulding us, into the person we are today, by the way we are affected by them. I am grateful for everyone I have ever met and all they have taught me and helped me to grow into the person I am today. For without them I would have never known about love, laughter, hurt, pain, sadness, anger and appreciation for another human being!

How every individual reacts to different situations and deals with their emotions, how they react to others or themselves, says a lot about the person they are. Most issues are stirred by the behaviors of others, with some type of reaction to what we believe to be our truth. These truths have been formulated by others over the years and the question I would ask you, 'does it feel right to you?' If you actually sit with what ever it is you have reacted too, in such a way that it has upset you, ask your self why?

Where did you first hear about it, see about it, even

read about it and how does it fit with what is true for you.

In my experience, if it doesn't feel right, feel good within me that I don't give it another thought.

If it plays on my mind, doesn't feel good then it is not what I believe to be true for me. Over the last couple of years I have had to completely start again of what I believe in because it shapes my entire life. 'Your beliefs are the blueprints of your life', they shape and mould your life and what you believe in manifests in any given form every single day.

How you feel is not only formulated by the thoughts you have but also you can pick up on how others are feeling too!

Your skin is the biggest sensory organ and detects how others are feeling through the vibrations they give off.

If you remember, everything gives off a certain amount of energy and depending on how you are feeling depends on the frequency of that vibration. We all pick up on the vibrations of, sadness, happiness, anger even hunger! How do you know whether the thoughts or feelings that you have are yours? Ask your body!

The same principle applies when muscle testing your body on what it would like to eat or drink.

You can muscle test yourself to see if that feeling is yours or someone else's. If you muscle test yourself every day it becomes second nature and you won't have to rock backwards or forwards, it will be like intuition. You will know, it will be the first thought that comes into your head. Trust that inner voice, that inner knowing which has always been there, but we were never taught how to use it!

I have been asking my body anything that has to do with it, food, clothes, feelings, healing, everything that involves my body I muscle test first.

It makes life so much easier, I am healthier, feel amazing and look great.

To help my body recover from losing a huge amount of weight, I have done many things from seeing a chiropractor, which I would never do before. Going and having massages was also a big step for me, letting someone else touch me, having acupuncture and going to Yoga.

Most of these were firsts for me, as I changed my views, so did my body and what it required for it to

move on to the next stage of rejuvenation. Your body is amazing and is capable of so much more than we realise, if we believe that it is possible, then anything can happen. People have cured themselves from cancer, walked again, life long diseases have disappeared all by changing how they think and believing it with every molecule of their being!
I knew there was more to life, I knew that my body was capable of more. I knew my body could heal it self, I just had to change from knowing to believing, trusting and listening to my body to make it possible! If I can do it, so can you!

HELP

Where are you?

I am calling you

Where are you?

You can not see me

Where are you?

You can not hear me

You are nowhere to be found

So I will wait for you

Until you come a calling

I will wait for you until your need is so great

I will wait for you until you ask that question

Then I will not hesitate

I will be there in a second

I will be there in a flash

I am here ready and waiting

Hoping and praying that you know

I am still here, while you are contemplating

Whether or not to ask

Will I hear you if you do

Will I help you if at all?

Please know that when you ask

No matter when

No matter where

No matter what

I am here to help you, always and forever more.

By Cheri Ann Revill

Letting Go

The rain is coming down in sheets covering the ground completely and everything else that lies in its wake. Water running down the plains, the mountains, the hills, the roads in rivulets going into the places that need it. Cleansing all that stand out in the open, feeling the droplets against their leaves, bark, fur, hair, skin, shells. Flowing over them, through them, washing away what once was so that they may start again with renewed vigor.

A real good soaking the earth is receiving, renewing its abundance ready for the rays of sun to poke its way through to kiss the earth, so everything may grow with new vitality to gift to us all what we require to live here comfortably. This planet provides all that live upon her, their daily requirements to live comfortably. Without the sun and the rain none of this would be possible!

People come and people go about their daily lives. Some may look up, others never do. So engrossed with what is going on within them, they may never be open to the possibilities that surround them.

Busy lives, busy minds, busy bodies not until they are

made to stop one way or another, that they wonder where their life has gone. If only they stopped to look around and enjoy what they already had instead of working to try and find what was missing. Life is here to be enjoyed, to be lived, but that seems to be forgotten as lives have progressed. I wish children were taught to enjoy their life, do what makes them happy, teach them that they are amazing beings and capable of incredible things! You are Happy, Healthy and Whole already, just stay like that for the rest of your life by believing that you already are!

That is my wish!

The idea behind letting go is metaphorically speaking! Letting go of fears, ideas, judgments, points of views that you may have had in areas of your life, that may not necessarily be working for you anymore.

Friendships change as time goes on, especially if you are changing and growing, others may not understand what is going on and don't like the change, that is OK! You are doing this for you, not for them. You may find other people will come into your life that see things the way you do, the way you think and feel.

It is good to have people that will support you and encourage your growth along your journey. There are friends, ones that you have known for many years, you may feel a sense of loyalty to. The things you used to have in common with them may start to change. I have a number of friends that I have known for over twenty years and I am extremely loyal to them. What I found, as I started to change, was with these friends, I had less and less contact with. Some I have not heard from for a few of years and others I get a message saying Hi, How are you doing?

This works well for where I am going and I am happy for them, I wish them all the best. In my experience I have found that when things start to change for you, many of your friends and family become confused with the changes happening within you and struggle to accept the change. As time passes, different people have come into my life that are supportive and like minded, which is very helpful for me as we all need that love and support from other people which helps us feel good.

As for relationships, I know my next love will be completely different because I have changed how I see myself, how I treat myself, I enjoy my own company and I know what kind of partner I would like to have.

I am very grateful for my children's father, we have four beautiful healthy children, two grandchildren and I have many wonderful memories from my marriage with him. By having that time to find myself, learn what I love to do, love myself and love my company, it has made a difference to how I view relationships and what I would like in a partner.

From what I have seen with others going into relationships straight after a separation, some work, some don't, as the relationship is similar to the one before, that didn't work for them.

There are many reasons for not wanting to be alone, not liking who they are, for financial reasons and many others. For me I did not want this to happen and I am glad I have taken the time for myself, I also didn't want to date, I want to be courted, as I felt there was a stigma around the whole dating scene.

My beliefs are different and everyone will have a different point of view on relationships and what they would like. I am happy, happy with myself, my life and I would like to find someone who has a similar feeling, I don't feel the need to make them happy and they me.

I found that to be one of the challenges in any relationship, one feels the need to make the other person in the relationship happy or show them their good points, their beauty. All you need to find out about yourself is within you. Love yourself unconditionally and you will find that loving another for who they are will come with ease.

What are you doing that you have been doing for so long that it has become a habit now? It could be something that you no longer like doing? Anything that doesn't feel good anymore? There are many different perceptions on what letting go means to an individual.

Firstly, for me, it was to stop living in the past and to let go of everything that had happened, that still affected me. Forgiving those who I felt had caused me hurt and pain, they may never even know they had but, it is a process for me I had to go through.

Then forgiving myself, this is a whole different realm of processing, because it means accepting responsibility for everything that has happened, the choices I made and to stop blaming myself for them.

For some it may be hard to get your head around this idea. In my experience this helped me to let go of all that happened in the past, the physical, and emotional abuse I had suffered, to change myself, knowing that it will never happen again! How do you change your self so that it doesn't happen again?

You may have seen time and again people go into the same relationships that don't work and they think there is something wrong with them. The choices they make are because of the way they feel about them selves. So to change how you feel about your self you need to look at your self in a different light and by doing that you need to wipe all that has happened in the past and start again. Look at your self from within, what do you like about yourself, what don't you like and why?

The judgment's you have about yourself you have seen, been told or heard, somewhere along the line and taken them on board as truth. Learn to like yourself, like your company, if you don't like your own company how can someone else enjoy your company? Love yourself, like you would like others to love you. It is something you have to work at every day and in my experience it has worked for me, it took some time but I got there eventually! I didn't like my own company, I didn't love me for who I was and once I started to do that everything else changed.

How I looked, how I treated myself and how others treated me! You put just as much energy into positive thoughts a you do, negative ones which creates the outcomes. I would rather have a happy, easy approach to life than the other way around. Yes, it is possible! Anything is possible, all you have to do is believe!

HUG

A hug is what is needed

A hug will get you far

A hug can make you forget everything

A hug can shift a star

A hug is something beautiful

A hug is always free

A hug is more than wonderful

A hug is definitely for Me

A hug can feed your soul

A hug can heal your heart

A hug is what is wanted

A hug now please is a start!

By Cheri Ann Revill

ABOUT THE AUTHOR

Cheri Ann Revill Author (A Journey of Self Love), Public Speaker, Innergetic Coach and Founder of Happiness with Ease
Mother of four children and Grandmother, lives in New South Wales, Australia.
On a Journey to find Happiness after a life once known crumbled after 23 years.

www.ingramcontent.com/pod-product-compliance
Lightning Source LLC
Chambersburg PA
CBHW071237280526
45787CB00002B/960